TYPE 2 DIABETES COOKBOOK

QUICK & EASY

60 Diabetic-Friendly Low Carb, Low Sugar, Low Fat,
High Protein Chicken, Beef, Pork,
Lamb and Vegetarian Recipes
that are done in 45 minutes or less

STELLA LAYNE

&

SELENA LANCASTER

CONTENT

PORK RECIPES

SEAFOOD RECIPES

VEGETARIAN RECIPES

NUTRITION SUMMARY   62

GRILLED LEMONGRASS BEEF

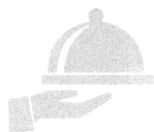

	SERVES		PREP TIME		COOK TIME
	2		**5** MINUTES		**15** MINUTES

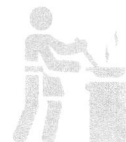

- **6 ounces** lean flank steak, thinly sliced

- **2 tablespoons** cup chopped lemongrass

- **1 clove** garlic, minced

- **1/2** serrano pepper, seeded and chopped

- **1 teaspoon** stevia

- **1/4 teaspoon** fish sauce

1. Preheat the broiler.

2. Blend lemongrass, garlic, pepper, stevia and fish sauce. Coat the steak in half the sauce and thread onto skewers. Broil for 12-15 minutes, turning occasionally.

3. While the meat is broiling, heat the remaining sauce in a sauce pan and thin with water if necessary. Pour the sauce on the skewer and serve.

CALORIES	CARBS	SUGAR	FAT	PROTEIN	SODIUM
124 KCAL	**3.6** GRAMS	**0.1** GRAMS	**3.8** GRAMS	**18.3** GRAMS	**182** MILLIGRAMS

MUSTARD BEEF LETTUCE WRAP

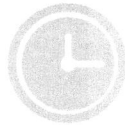

	SERVES 3		PREP TIME 5 MINUTES		COOK TIME 15 MINUTES

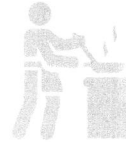

1. Brown the steak over medium heat.

2. Slice the carrot and cucumber lengthwise to form strips

3. Evenly divide beef, carrot and cucumber on each lettuce leave. Spread the Dijonnaise on top then roll up.

- **6 ounces** lean top round steak, finely cubed

- **6** Romaine lettuce leaves

- **1** medium carrot, peeled

- **1** large cucumber, peeled

- **3 tablespoons** Dijonnaise

- Nonstick Cooking Spray

CALORIES	CARBS	SUGAR	FAT	PROTEIN	SODIUM
155 KCAL	5.8 GRAMS	2.5 GRAMS	3.8 GRAMS	21.0 GRAMS	227 MILLIGRAMS

BEEF AND VEGGIE STIR FRY

	SERVES 2		PREP TIME 15 MINUTES		COOK TIME 10 MINUTES

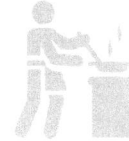

- **1/2 pound** lean flank steak, cut into strips

- **2 tablespoons** fat-free beef broth

- **1 cup** broccoli florets

- **1/2 cup** sliced bell peppers

- **1/2 cup** sliced carrot

- **1** green onion, chopped

- **1 clove** garlic, minced

- **1 tablespoon** low sodium soy sauce

- **1/2 tablespoon** grated ginger

- **1/2 teaspoon** stevia

1. In a small bowl, mix beef with soy sauce, stevia and ginger. Set aside to marinate for 10 minutes.

2. Spray a large skillet. Sauté the onion until fragrant. Then add all the vegetables. Cook for 4-5 minutes until vegetables are tender. Remove from the skillet.

3. Add the beef. Reserve the marinade. Cook until the beef is brown. Then return the vegetables, broth and marinade. Stir and cook for 2 minutes.

CALORIES	CARBS	SUGAR	FAT	PROTEIN	SODIUM
198 KCAL	9.2 GRAMS	3.8 GRAMS	5.2 GRAMS	26.8 GRAMS	674 MILLIGRAMS

QUICK TACO AND BEANS SOUP

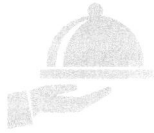

	SERVES		PREP TIME		COOK TIME
	6		**5** MINUTES		**25** MINUTES

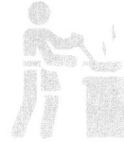

1. In a non-stick pan, sauté the beef until brown over medium heat. Drain the excess oil.

2. Place all ingredients in a stock pot. Bring the soup to a boil then reduce to low heat and simmer for 10 minutes.

3. Serve the soup with the fat-free ranch dressing on top.

- **1/2 pound** 95% lean ground beef
- **1 package** of taco seasoning
- **1 ounce** fat-free ranch dressing
- **1** 10.5-ounce **can** kidney beans, undrained
- **1** 10.5-ounce **can** pinto beans, undrained
- **1** 10.5-ounce **can** black beans, undrained
- **1 cup** crushed tomatoes

CALORIES	CARBS	SUGAR	FAT	PROTEIN	SODIUM
216 KCAL	**29.2** GRAMS	**2.8** GRAMS	**2.2** GRAMS	**20.0** GRAMS	**536** MILLIGRAMS

ONE-PAN MEXICAN BEEF

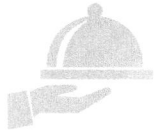

SERVES **2**	PREP TIME **10** MINUTES	COOK TIME **35** MINUTES

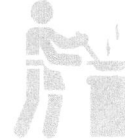

- **1/2 pound** lean flank steak, cut into strips
- **1/2 cup** sliced onion
- **1/2 cup** sliced mushroom
- **1/2 cup** sliced red bell pepper
- **6 tablespoons** fat-free low sodium chicken broth
- **1/4 cup** no-sugar-added salsa
- **1 clove** garlic, minced
- **1 teaspoon** chili powder
- **1/2 teaspoon** paprika
- **1/4 teaspoon** salt
- Nonstick Cooking Spray

1. In a medium bowl, season the beef with chili powder, salt and paprika.

2. Spray a large skillet, cook the beef for 3 minutes. Set aside.

3. Sauté the garlic, onion and bell peppers until fragrant. Then add mushroom and cook for another 2 minutes.

4. Add broth and salsa. Simmer until the liquid is reduced by half. Stir in beef and cook for 1 minute.

CALORIES	CARBS	SUGAR	FAT	PROTEIN	SODIUM
204 KCAL	**8.8** GRAMS	**3.8** GRAMS	**5.4** GRAMS	**26.4** GRAMS	**678** MILLIGRAMS

GREEK SPINACH CHICKEN SALAD

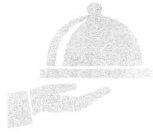

	SERVES		PREP TIME		COOK TIME
	3		5 MINUTES		10 MINUTES

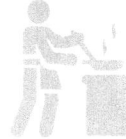

1. In a medium bowl, combine yogurt, lemon juice and seasoning

2. In a large bowl, mix all ingredients except spinach.

3. Serve with spinach.

- **1 can** 12.5-ounce chicken breast, drained
- **2 cups** baby spinach leaves
- **1** medium tomato, sliced
- **1/2 cup** chopped bell pepper
- **1/2 cup** fat-free Greek yogurt
- **1/4 cup** chopped cilantro
- **2 tablespoons** sliced almond
- **1 teaspoon** lemon juice
- **1 teaspoon** curry powder
- **1/4 teaspoon** salt
- **1/8 teaspoon** ground black pepper

CALORIES	CARBS	SUGAR	FAT	PROTEIN	SODIUM
180 KCAL	11.8 GRAMS	6.2 GRAMS	6.0 GRAMS	27.6 GRAMS	452 MILLIGRAMS

RANCH CHICKEN SALAD

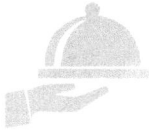

	SERVES 3		PREP TIME 5 MINUTES		COOK TIME 10 MINUTES

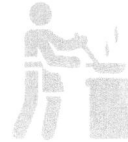

- **1 can** 12.5-ounce chicken breast, drained

- **1/2 cup** chopped bell peppers

- **1/4 cup** chopped green onion

- **1 1/2 tablespoons** fat-free mayonnaise

- **1 tablespoon** light ranch dressing

- **1 tablespoon** lemon juice

- **1/4 teaspoon** ground black pepper

1. In a small bowl, combine mayonnaise, ranch dressing, lemon juice and pepper

2. In a large bowl, toss all ingredients together and serve.

CALORIES	CARBS	SUGAR	FAT	PROTEIN	SODIUM
126 KCAL	10.0 GRAMS	5.6 GRAMS	3.4 GRAMS	20.2 GRAMS	630 MILLIGRAMS

LENTIL TURKEY SAUSAGE

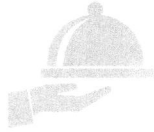

	SERVES 6		PREP TIME 5 MINUTES		COOK TIME 10 MINUTES

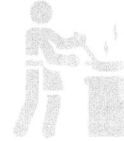

1. In a small bowl, mix the flaxseed meal and egg white. Set aside.

2. In a medium pot, add lentil and cover with water by 1-inch. Bring it to boil and cook for 15 minutes. Drain the lentils and mash well.

3. In a large bowl, combine all ingredients.

4. Divide the mixture into 12 portions and shape into patties.

5. Spray a non-stick pan. Heat the patties for 3-5 minutes over low/medium heat until brown. Flip and heat for another 3-5 minutes.

- 12 ounce extra lean ground turkey
- 1 cup chopped onion
- 1/2 cup dry red lentils
- 1/4 cup sliced black olives
- 3 tablespoons liquid egg whites
- 1/4 cup fat-free mozzarella cheese
- 1/4 cup low-fat parmesan cheese
- 6 tablespoons whole-wheat breadcrumbs
- 2 tablespoons flax seed meal
- 1/2 teaspoon salt
- 1/4 teaspoon pepper
- Nonstick Cooking Spray

CALORIES	CARBS	SUGAR	FAT	PROTEIN	SODIUM
192 KCAL	19.2 GRAMS	1.8 GRAMS	2.6 GRAMS	22.2 GRAMS	392 MILLIGRAMS

HERB ROASTED CHICKEN

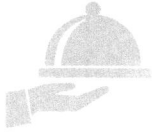

	SERVES 2		PREP TIME 5 MINUTES		COOK TIME 15 MINUTES

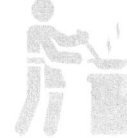

- **6 ounces** boneless skinless chicken breast

- **1 teaspoon** olive oil

- **1/4 teaspoon** garlic powder

- **1/4 teaspoon** dried basil

- **1/4 teaspoon** dried rosemary

- **1/4 teaspoon** dried thyme

- **1/8 teaspoon** salt

1. Preheat the broiler

2. In a small bowl, combine oil, herbs and seasoning.

3. Coat the chicken evenly. Broil for 12-15 minutes. Flip once.

CALORIES	CARBS	SUGAR	FAT	PROTEIN	SODIUM
105	0.5	0.0	4.5	16.6	315
KCAL	GRAMS	GRAMS	GRAMS	GRAMS	MILLIGRAMS

SPICY CITRUS CHICKEN STIR FRY

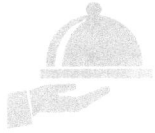

	SERVES	PREP TIME	COOK TIME
	2	**10** MINUTES	**10** MINUTES

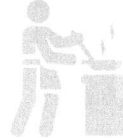

1. In a small bowl, combine lime juice, hot sauce, soy sauce and all spices.

2. Add sesame oil to a non-stick sauce pan and sauté garlic for 1 minutes. Add in shrimp and sauté until pink.

3. Add the sauce. Stir to coat the shrimp evenly and heat until sauce is bubbly.

- **6 ounces** boneless skinless chicken breast, sliced
- **1 clove** garlic, minced
- **1 teaspoon** lime juice
- **1/2 teaspoon** sesame oil
- **1/2 teaspoon** hot sauce
- **1/4 teaspoon** low-sodium soy sauce
- **1/8 teaspoon** ground coriander
- **1/8 teaspoon** red pepper flakes
- Pinch of ground ginger

CALORIES	CARBS	SUGAR	FAT	PROTEIN	SODIUM
98 KCAL	**0.5** GRAMS	**0.1** GRAMS	**3.4** GRAMS	**16.6** GRAMS	**239** MILLIGRAMS

CHICKEN FAJITA

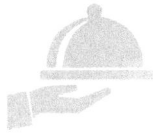

	SERVES 4		PREP TIME 10 MINUTES		COOK TIME 10 MINUTES

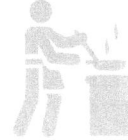

- **1 pound** boneless skinless chicken breast, sliced

- **1** green bell pepper, cut into strips

- **1** small onion, cut into strips

- **2 cloves** garlic, minced

- **1 tablespoon** lemon juice

- **1 teaspoon** ground coriander

- **1 teaspoon** dried oregano

- **1/2 teaspoon** ground ginger

- **1/2 teaspoon** cumin

- **1/2 teaspoon** paprika

- **1/4 teaspoon** salt

1. Spray a non-stick sauce pan and sauté chicken with salt and pepper until cooked through. Then add onion, bell peppers and sauté until soft.

2. Add lemon juice, all herbs and spices. Sauté for another 2 minutes. Serve immediately.

CALORIES	CARBS	SUGAR	FAT	PROTEIN	SODIUM
134 KCAL	4.1 GRAMS	0.9 GRAMS	3.3 GRAMS	22.7 GRAMS	375 MILLIGRAMS

TRADITIONAL TURKEY SAUSAGE

	SERVES		PREP TIME		COOK TIME
	4		**5** MINUTES		**15** MINUTES

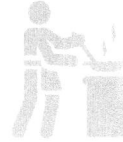

1. In a medium bowl, Combine all ingredients. Divide the mixture into 8 portions and shape into 1/2-inch thick patties.

2. Spray a non-stick pan and heat over medium heat. Add the patties and cook for 4-5 minutes then flip and cooked for another 4-5 minutes or until golden brown.

- **1 pound** 93% lean ground turkey
- **1 teaspoon** fennel seed
- **1 teaspoon** ground black pepper
- **1 teaspoon** sage
- **1 teaspoon** ground thyme
- **1/2 teaspoon** garlic powder
- **1/2 teaspoon** onion power
- **1/2 teaspoon** salt
- **1/4 teaspoon** ground nutmeg

CALORIES	CARBS	SUGAR	FAT	PROTEIN	SODIUM
158 KCAL	**1.6** GRAMS	**0.0** GRAMS	**8.2** GRAMS	**22.2** GRAMS	**380** MILLIGRAMS

CHICKEN AND PEAS STIR FRY

	SERVES **2**		PREP TIME **10** MINUTES		COOK TIME **15** MINUTES

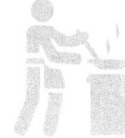

- **1/2 pound** chicken tender, cut into strips

- **6 ounces** sugar snap peas, cut into strips

- **1/2 tablespoon** oyster sauce

- **1 clove** garlic, minced

- **1** green onion, chopped

- salt and pepper to taste

1. Spray a large skillet. Brown the chicken. Add oyster sauce and cook for another minute. Set aside.

2. Sauté green onion and garlic until fragrant. Then add peas and cook until fragrant. Stir in chicken and stir-fry for 30 seconds.

CALORIES **118** KCAL	CARBS **3.4** GRAMS	SUGAR **1.2** GRAMS	FAT **0.6** GRAMS	PROTEIN **23.0** GRAMS	SODIUM **236** MILLIGRAMS

CAPRESE CHICKEN

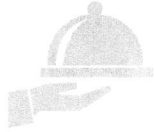

SERVES
6

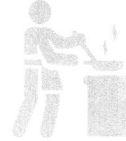

PREP TIME
10
MINUTES

COOK TIME
20
MINUTES

1. Heat a grill or a grill pan over moderate to moderately high heat.

2. Lightly pour 1 tablespoon of olive oil over chicken breasts and season to taste with pepper.

3. Sprinkle Italian seasoning over the chicken.

4. Place the chicken on the grill and cook for 3 to 5 minutes each side, or until cooked well. Cooking time will vary based on the thickness of your chicken breasts.

5. When chicken is cooked well, top with a slice of mozzarella cheese and cook for an additional minute to two minutes.

6. Remove from heat and place chicken breasts on a separate plate. Top each breast with one slice of tomato, thinly sliced basil and pepper to taste.

7. Season with balsamic vinegar or balsamic glaze and serve.

- **1 pound** boneless, skinless chicken breasts

- **1 tablespoon** olive oil

- **1 teaspoon** dry Italian seasoning (or equal parts of garlic powder, dried oregano and dried basil)

- **4** thick (½-inch) **slices** ripe tomato

- **4** 1-ounce **slices** fresh mozzarella cheese

- **3 tablespoons** balsamic vinegar

- **2 tablespoons** thinly sliced basil

- Pepper to taste

CALORIES	CARBS	SUGAR	FAT	PROTEIN	SODIUM
153	**2.7**	**1.2**	**4.0**	**22.0**	**70**
KCAL	GRAMS	GRAMS	GRAMS	GRAMS	MILLIGRAMS

WHITE BEAN AND CHICKEN SOUP

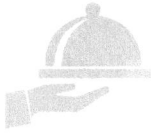

SERVES	PREP TIME	COOK TIME
6	10 MINUTES	20 MINUTES

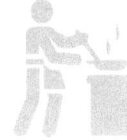

- **1 pound** boneless skinless chicken breast, diced

- **1** leek, chopped

- **1** small onion, chopped

- **1 can** 15-ounce cannellini beans, rinsed and drained

- **2 cups** fat-free low sodium chicken broth

- **1 tablespoon** chopped fresh sage

- **1 tablespoon** chopped fresh dill

- **1 teaspoon** chopped fresh rosemary

- **1** bay leave

- **1/4 teaspoon** salt

1. Spray a large pot. Sauté leek and onion over medium heat until softened.

2. Add broth and 2 cups of water. Bring it to a boil. Then add all other ingredients. Heat for 5-10 minutes.

CALORIES	CARBS	SUGAR	FAT	PROTEIN	SODIUM
160 KCAL	16.0 GRAMS	1.6 GRAMS	2.2 GRAMS	20.2 GRAMS	610 MILLIGRAMS

CHICKEN AND AVOCADO LETTUCE WRAP

	SERVES		PREP TIME		COOK TIME
	2		5 MINUTES		25 MINUTES

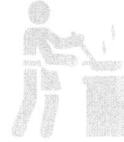

1. In a medium bowl, mix chicken, avocadoes, tomatoes and dressing together

2. Evenly divide the filling onto each lettuce leave and roll up.

- **8 ounces** boneless skinless chicken breast, cooked and shredded

- 8 Romaine lettuce leaves

- **1/2** medium avocado, chopped

- **1/4 cup** light Italian dressing

- **1/4 cup** chopped tomatoes

CALORIES	CARBS	SUGAR	FAT	PROTEIN	SODIUM
216 KCAL	10.6 GRAMS	3.2 GRAMS	9.2 GRAMS	23.6 GRAMS	542 MILLIGRAMS

TURKEY SATAY

 **SERVES**
6

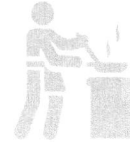 **PREP TIME**
10
MINUTES

COOK TIME
20
MINUTES

- **1 pound** turkey breast, diced

- **1 cup** low-fat coconut milk

- **2 cloves** garlic, minced

- **3 tablespoons** powdered peanut butter

- **1 tablespoon** Truvia brown sugar

- **1 teaspoon** turmeric

- **1/4 teaspoon** salt

1. Preheat broiler.

2. Thread the turkey onto 12 skewers.

3. In a small bowl, combine all other ingredients. Coat the skewer with the half of the sauce. Set aside to marinade for 10 minutes. Then broil for 10-15 minutes or until crispy.

4. While the meat is broiling, heat the remaining sauce in a pan. Pour over the skewer and serve.

CALORIES	CARBS	SUGAR	FAT	PROTEIN	SODIUM
126	**18.4**	**3.7**	**5.4**	**3.4**	**406**
KCAL	GRAMS	GRAMS	GRAMS	GRAMS	MILLIGRAMS

LEMON AND THYME CHICKEN

	SERVES		PREP TIME		COOK TIME
	2		**15** MINUTES		**20** MINUTES

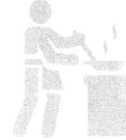

1. In a large bowl, mix the chicken in all other ingredients. Set aside to marinate for 15 minutes.

2. Spray a large skillet. Cook the chicken until cook through, about 4-5 minutes each side

- **1/2 pound** chicken tender

- **2 tablespoons** lemon juice

- **3 sprigs** fresh thyme, chopped

- **1/2 tablespoon** lemon zest

- **1 clove** garlic, minced

- salt and pepper to taste

- Nonstick Cooking Spray

CALORIES	CARBS	SUGAR	FAT	PROTEIN	SODIUM
110 KCAL	**2.0** GRAMS	**0.4** GRAMS	**0.4** GRAMS	**22.6** GRAMS	**112** MILLIGRAMS

SPINACH FETA STUFFED CHICKEN

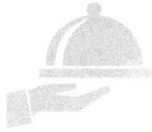

	SERVES 2	PREP TIME 10 MINUTES	COOK TIME 25 MINUTES

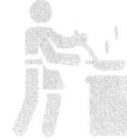

- **2** boneless, skinless chicken breast, flattened
- **5 ounces** frozen spinach, thawed and squeeze
- **1/4 cup** fat-free feta cheese
- **3 tablespoons** fat-free ricotta cheese
- **2 tablespoons** chopped green onion
- **2 tablespoons** chopped fresh parsley
- **1/2 tablespoon** fresh dill
- **1 clove** garlic
- salt and pepper to taste

1. Preheat the oven to 350°F.

2. Spray a large skillet.

3. Sauté the green onion and garlic until fragrant. Add spinach, parsley and dill. Cool until heated through. Season with salt and pepper.

4. Remove from heat and stir in feta cheese and ricotta cheese.

5. Divide the mixture onto the chicken breast. Roll up. Rub the chicken with salt and pepper.

6. Bake for 25 minutes.

CALORIES	CARBS	SUGAR	FAT	PROTEIN	SODIUM
166 KCAL	4.2 GRAMS	1.6 GRAMS	1.2 GRAMS	30.0 GRAMS	656 MILLIGRAMS

FOOL-PROOF SALSA CHICKEN

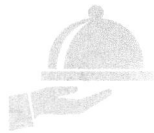

	SERVES 2		PREP TIME 5 MINUTES		COOK TIME 35 MINUTES

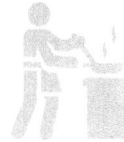

1. Preheat the oven to 350°F.

2. Season the chicken with half of the taco seasoning.

3. Brown the chicken in an -oven-proof skillet. Then stir in salsa and the remaining seasoning.

4. Cover and bake for 30 minutes.

5. Shred the chicken and stir in sour cream.

- **1/2 pound** chicken tender
- **1 cup** salsa
- **1/2 package** taco seasoning
- **1/2 cup** fat-free soup cream
- Nonstick Cooking Spray

CALORIES	CARBS	SUGAR	FAT	PROTEIN	SODIUM
184 KCAL	11.0 GRAMS	8.0 GRAMS	0.4 GRAMS	24.0 GRAMS	292 MILLIGRAMS

PINTO BEAN TURKEY ENCHILADAS

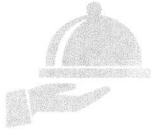

	SERVES 4	PREP TIME 10 MINUTES	COOK TIME 30 MINUTES

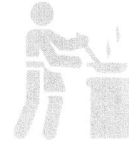

- **6** medium scallions, white and green parts chopped

- **12 ounces** 93% ground turkey. Sautéed until slightly brown.

- **12 ounces** canned low sodium pinto beans, drained and rinsed

- **1 cup** canned enchilada sauce or taco sauce, divided

- **4** medium-sized low-carb tortillas

- **1/4 cup** shredded reduced fat Mexican cheese

1. Preheat oven to 350 degrees.

2. Mix scallions, turkey, beans, and ½ cup enchilada or taco sauce.

3. Fill each tortilla with ¼ of turkey-bean mixture. Fold in sides, top and bottom of tortilla to completely enclose the filling inside the tortilla.

4. Place tortillas seam side down in a 9x13-inch baking dish.

5. Pour the remaining ½ cup of sauce over top of enchiladas and add the cheese.

6. Cover pan and bake until heated through and cheese is hot and bubbly (about 20 minutes).

CALORIES	CARBS	SUGAR	FAT	PROTEIN	SODIUM
288 KCAL	21.0 GRAMS	0.0 GRAMS	9.6 GRAMS	22.8 GRAMS	650 MILLIGRAMS

POMODORO CHICKEN WITH SQUASH

SERVES	PREP TIME	COOK TIME
4	20 MINUTES	20 MINUTES

1. In a non-stick sauce pan, add oil and sauté chicken with seasoning until cooked through. Then add garlic and onion sauté for 2 minutes.

2. Stir in tomatoes and bring the mixture to a boil. Reduce to low heat and simmer for 5-10 minutes to reduce.

3. Toss in squash noodles and heat for 3-4 minutes or until the desired texture is reached. Sprinkle with basil and serve.

- **1/2** medium butternut squash, seeded and spiralized

- **12 ounces** boneless skinless chicken breast, diced

- **1 can** 14.5-ounce crushed tomatoes

- **1/2 cup** chopped onion

- **1 clove** garlic, minced

- **1 1/2 tablespoons** chopped basil

- **1/4 teaspoon** salt

- **1/8 teaspoon** ground black pepper

CALORIES	CARBS	SUGAR	FAT	PROTEIN	SODIUM
182 KCAL	9.5 GRAMS	0.9 GRAMS	2.6 GRAMS	18.5 GRAMS	452 MILLIGRAMS

CHICKEN BASQUE WITH ZUCCHINI NOODLE

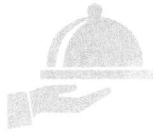

	SERVES 2		PREP TIME 20 MINUTES		COOK TIME 20 MINUTES

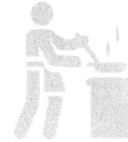

- **1** medium zucchini, spiralized

- **6 ounces** boneless skinless chicken breast, diced

- **1/2 cup** grape tomatoes, quartered

- **1/4 cup** thinly sliced red bell peppers

- **1/4 cup** chopped yellow onion

- **1/4 cup** fat-free low sodium chicken broth

- **1 tablespoon** chopped fresh parsley

- **1/4 teaspoon** fresh thyme

- **1/8 teaspoon** paprika

- **1/8 teaspoon** red pepper flakes

- **1/8 teaspoon** salt

1. In a non-stick sauce pan, add oil and sauté chicken with salt until cooked through. Then add paprika, bell peppers and onion sauté for 2 minutes.

2. Add tomatoes, broth, thyme, red pepper flakes and bring the mixture to a boil. Reduce to low heat and simmer for 5-10 minutes to reduce.

3. Toss in zoodles and heat for 2-3 minutes or until the desired texture is reached. Sprinkle with parsley and serve.

CALORIES	CARBS	SUGAR	FAT	PROTEIN	SODIUM
113 KCAL	8.6 GRAMS	5.9 GRAMS	2.6 GRAMS	18.9 GRAMS	372 MILLIGRAMS

THAI CHICKEN ZOODLES

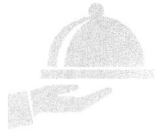

	SERVES		PREP TIME		COOK TIME
	2		20 MINUTES		20 MINUTES

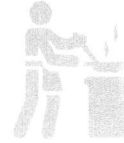

1. In a small bowl, combine powdered peanut butter, soy sauce, chilli paste and syrup.

2. In a large bowl, toss all ingredients together and serve.

- 1 medium zucchini, spiralized
- **6 ounces** boneless skinless chicken breast, diced
- **2 tablespoons** powdered peanut butter
- **1 tablespoon** dry roasted peanuts, crushed
- **1 teaspoon** low sodium soy sauce
- **1/2 teaspoon** chilli garlic paste
- **1/2 teaspoon** Truvia Nectar / Stevia Syrup

CALORIES	CARBS	SUGAR	FAT	PROTEIN	SODIUM
141 KCAL	6.8 GRAMS	3.6 GRAMS	4.8 GRAMS	20.1 GRAMS	363 MILLIGRAMS

HAWAIIAN TUNA POKE

	SERVES 2	PREP TIME 5 MINUTES	COOK TIME 5 MINUTES

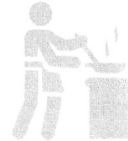

- **1/2 pound** sushi grade tuna, cubed

- **1/4 cup** finely chopped green onion

- **2 tablespoons** low sodium soy sauce

- **1 teaspoon** lime juice

- **1 teaspoon** roasted sesame seed

1. In a medium bowl, combine all ingredients and serve.

CALORIES	CARBS	SUGAR	FAT	PROTEIN	SODIUM
182 KCAL	2.0 GRAMS	0.0 GRAMS	4.8 GRAMS	29.4 GRAMS	620 MILLIGRAMS

TUNA SALAD LETTUCE WRAPS

	SERVES		PREP TIME		COOK TIME
	2		5 MINUTES		5 MINUTES

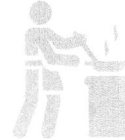

1. In a medium bowl, mix tuna, yogurt, salt and pepper. Adjust seasoning if needed.

2. Evenly divide the filling onto the lettuce leaves and roll up.

- 1 5-ounce **can** tuna packed in water, drained
- **3 ounces** fat-free Greek Yogurt
- 4 Romaine Lettuce Leaves
- **1/8 teaspoon** salt
- **1/8 teaspoon** pepper

CALORIES	CARBS	SUGAR	FAT	PROTEIN	SODIUM
95 KCAL	4.8 GRAMS	1.8 GRAMS	1.4 GRAMS	17.3 GRAMS	388 MILLIGRAMS

CURRY SPICED SALMON STEAK

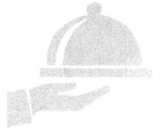

SERVES 2	PREP TIME 10 MINUTES	COOK TIME 10 MINUTES

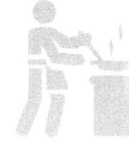

- **2** salmon fillets (6-ounce each)
- **1 teaspoon** curry powder
- **1 teaspoon** garlic powder
- **1/2 teaspoon** cumin
- **1/4 teaspoon** salt

1. Preheat the broiler.

2. Mix the spice in a small bowl. Rub the spice evenly on the salmon.

3. Broil for 8-12 minutes.

CALORIES	CARBS	SUGAR	FAT	PROTEIN	SODIUM
160 KCAL	1.8 GRAMS	0.0 GRAMS	1.8 GRAMS	36.4 GRAMS	512 MILLIGRAMS

SIMPLE RAINBOW TROUT

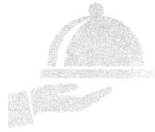

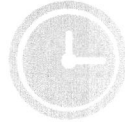

	SERVES 2		PREP TIME 5 MINUTES		COOK TIME 15 MINUTES

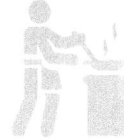

1. Clean and rinse fish fillets. Check to make sure that all bones are removed. Pat dry.

2. In a separate container, mix the cornmeal, salt, pepper, celery seed and chopped parsley.

3. Cover fish with cornmeal mixture and press onto fish fillets.

4. Heat olive oil in non-stick skillet. Cook fish 2 to 3 minutes per side. Fish should be brown and crisp and should flake when pierced with a fork or a knife.

- **8 ounces** rainbow trout fillets
- **3 tablespoons** yellow cornmeal
- **1 1/3 tablespoons** chopped parsley
- **2 teaspoons** olive oil
- **1/4 teaspoon** ground celery seeds
- **1/4 teaspoon** ground black pepper
- **1 pinch** salt

CALORIES	CARBS	SUGAR	FAT	PROTEIN	SODIUM
240 KCAL	10.0 GRAMS	0.0 GRAMS	5.0 GRAMS	25.0 GRAMS	338 MILLIGRAMS

TUNA CAKE

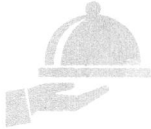

SERVES
2

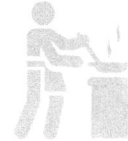

PREP TIME
5
MINUTES

COOK TIME
15
MINUTES

- **2** 3-ounce **cans** tuna, in water

- **2** egg whites

- **8** Wheat Thins crackers, crushed

- **2 tablespoons** grated carrot

- **2 tablespoons** chopped water chestnuts, capers or diced red pepper

- **1/2 tablespoon** minced onion, if tolerated

- Pepper, dill and dried mustard, to taste

1. Mix all the ingredients together in a container.

2. Form mixture into eight patties with hands.

3. Spray medium-sized skillet with nonstick cooking spray and place over medium heat.

4. Cook patties until golden brown on both sides, 2-3 minutes per side.

CALORIES	CARBS	SUGAR	FAT	PROTEIN	SODIUM
160	8.0	0.0	2.0	24.0	480
KCAL	GRAMS	GRAMS	GRAMS	GRAMS	MILLIGRAMS

DIJON LEMON ORANGE ROUGHY

	SERVES	PREP TIME	COOK TIME
	2	5 MINUTES	15 MINUTES

1. Cover the rack of a broiler pan or a baking sheet with tin foil and spray foil with cooking spray.

2. Combine lemon juice, mustard, olive oil and ground pepper. Stir thoroughly.

3. Place fish fillets on rack or baking sheet.

4. Brush fillets with half the lemon juice mixture, and then set aside the remaining half.

5. Broil fish for 5 minutes or until fish flakes easily.

6. Drizzle the remaining lemon juice mixture over the fillets and add pepper.

7. Serve with lemon wedges.

- **1/2 pound** orange roughy fillets
- **8** medium lemon wedges
- **1 1/2 tablespoons** lemon juice
- **1/2 tablespoon** Dijon mustard
- **1/2 tablespoon** olive oil
- **1/8 teaspoon** ground pepper

CALORIES	CARBS	SUGAR	FAT	PROTEIN	SODIUM
228 KCAL	6.0 GRAMS	0.0 GRAMS	8.0 GRAMS	34.0 GRAMS	314 MILLIGRAMS

LEMONY TILAPIA

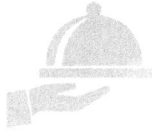

	SERVES		PREP TIME		COOK TIME
	1		5 MINUTES		15 MINUTES

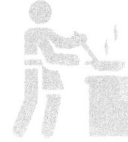

- **4 ounces** tilapia fillet
- **1/2 tablespoon** lemon juice
- **1/2 tablespoon** reduced fat or light mayonnaise
- **3/4 tablespoon** finely chopped green onions
- **1/4 teaspoon** dried basil
- A pinch of salt
- A pinch of Black pepper

1. Preheat oven to 350 °F.

2. Place the fillet in a buttered baking dish.

3. Sprinkle the top with lemon juice.

4. Bake fish in preheated oven 10 to 20 minutes or until fish starts to flake.

5. Meanwhile, mix the mayonnaise, onions and seasonings in a bowl using a fork.

6. When the fish is ready, spread the top with the mixture and bake until golden brown (approximately 5 minutes, depending on the thickness of the fish).

CALORIES	CARBS	SUGAR	FAT	PROTEIN	SODIUM
121 KCAL	1.3 GRAMS	0.3 GRAMS	4.3 GRAMS	20.1 GRAMS	282.3 MILLIGRAMS

SPICY CUTRUS TILAPIA

SERVES
2

PREP TIME
5
MINUTES

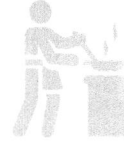

COOK TIME
15
MINUTES

1. Preheat the oven to 400°F.

2. In small bowl, combine lime juice, spice and seasoning.

3. Coat the fillet evenly with the sauce. Place the fillets in a baking sheet and cover with foil.

4. Bake for 10 minutes. Then remove the foil, change to broiler setting and broil for 2-5 minutes.

- **1/2 pound** tilapia fillets
- **1 tablespoon** lime juice
- **1/2 tablespoon** chilli powder
- **1/4 teaspoon** paprika
- **1/4 teaspoon** cumin
- **1/4 teaspoon** dried cayenne pepper
- **1/8 teaspoon** salt

CALORIES	CARBS	SUGAR	FAT	PROTEIN	SODIUM
134	25.3	3.4	1.5	0.3	294
KCAL	GRAMS	GRAMS	GRAMS	GRAMS	MILLIGRAMS

BROILED CITRUS SALMON

SERVES
2

PREP TIME
5
MINUTES

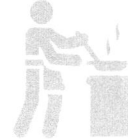

COOK TIME
20
MINUTES

- **2** salmon fillets (6-ounce each)
- **1** lemon, thinly sliced
- **2 tablespoons** lemon juice
- **1 tablespoon** lemon zest
- **3 cloves** garlic, minced
- **1 cup** fat-free low sodium chicken broth
- **2 tablespoons** chopped fresh parsley
- salt and pepper to taste
- Non-stick Cooking Spray

1. Brown the salmon fillet. Set aside.

2. Sauté garlic until fragrant.

3. Add lemon zest, lemon juice and broth. Simmer on low until reduces by half. Season with salt and pepper.

4. Return the Salmon. Simmer until the salmon is cooked through. Sprinkle parsley and serve.

CALORIES	CARBS	SUGAR	FAT	PROTEIN	SODIUM
166	3.6	0.4	1.6	37.4	264
KCAL	GRAMS	GRAMS	GRAMS	GRAMS	MILLIGRAMS

SALMON AND EGG SCRAMBLE

	SERVES 2		PREP TIME 10 MINUTES		COOK TIME 15 MINUTES

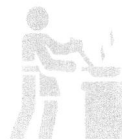

1. Sauté garlic and spinach until fragrant.

2. In a medium bowl, whisk the eggs and cheese. Season with salt and pepper.

3. Add the egg mixture. Scramble for 30 seconds.

4. Add salmon. Scramble for until eggs are cooked through.

- **4 ounces** smoked salmon
- **2** large eggs and **4** egg whites
- **2 cups** baby spinach
- **2 cloves** garlic, minced
- **2 tablespoons** low fat cheddar cheese
- salt and pepper to taste
- Nonstick Cooking Spray

CALORIES	CARBS	SUGAR	FAT	PROTEIN	SODIUM
194 KCAL	2.8 GRAMS	0.8 GRAMS	7.8 GRAMS	26.2 GRAMS	640 MILLIGRAMS

ITALIAN TILAPIA ALFREDO

SERVES 4

PREP TIME 5 MINUTES

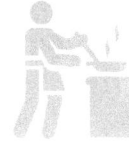

COOK TIME 20 MINUTES

- **1 pound** tilapia fillet, cut into 2-inch pieces
- **1 10.5-ounce can** fat-free condensed cream of mushroom soup
- **1 10-ounce can** diced tomatoes, drained
- **1/2 cup** chopped onion
- **3 cloves** garlic, minced
- **1/2 cup** skim milk
- **2 tablespoons** chopped fresh parsley
- salt and pepper to taste
- Nonstick Cooking Spray

1. Season the fish with salt and pepper. Set aside.

2. Sauté garlic and onion until fragrant.

3. Add soup, milk and tomatoes. Cook unti bubbly. Add Fish and bring it to a boil. Then reduce to low and simmer for 10-15 minutes.

CALORIES	CARBS	SUGAR	FAT	PROTEIN	SODIUM
168	11.6	3.6	4.2	22.6	648
KCAL	GRAMS	GRAMS	GRAMS	GRAMS	MILLIGRAMS

CHEESY SPICY HALIBUT

	SERVES		PREP TIME		COOK TIME
	2		**15** MINUTES		**10** MINUTES

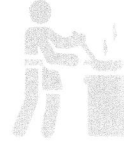

1. Preheat the oven to 425°F.

2. In a medium bowl, combine all ingredients except fish.

3. Season the fish with salt and pepper. Place the fish on a baking dish. Bake for 10 minutes.

4. Spread the cheese mixture on top and bake for another 5 minutes or until cheese are bubbly and golden brown.

- **1/2 pound** skinless halibut fillets

- **1** green onion, chopped

- **1/4 cup** fat-free parmesan cheese

- **2 teaspoons** fat-free mayonnaise

- **1/2 tablespoons** lemon juice

- **1/2 teaspoon** hot sauce

- **1/8 teaspoon** salt

- Nonstick Cooking Spray

CALORIES	CARBS	SUGAR	FAT	PROTEIN	SODIUM
136 KCAL	**7.6** GRAMS	**0.6** GRAMS	**1.0** GRAMS	**25.0** GRAMS	**540** MILLIGRAMS

MACKEREL CAKES

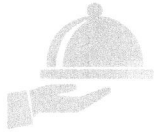

	SERVES 4	PREP TIME 5 MINUTES	COOK TIME 20 MINUTES

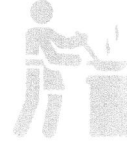

- **1 15-ounce can** Jack mackerel, drained
- **1/2 cup** rolled oats
- **6 tablespoons** liquid egg whites
- **1/2 cup** chopped onion
- **1/2 tablespoon** garlic powder
- **1/2 teaspoon** chilli powder
- **1/2 teaspoon** paprika
- **1/2 teaspoon** cumin seed
- **1/4 teaspoon** salt
- Nonstick Cooking Spray

1. Preheat the oven to 400°F.

2. In a large bowl, combine all ingredients.

3. Divide the mixture into 8 portions and shape into patties.

4. Spray the baking tray and the patties.

5. Bake for 15 minutes or until slightly brown, turning half-way through.

CALORIES	CARBS	SUGAR	FAT	PROTEIN	SODIUM
204 KCAL	9.6 GRAMS	1.2 GRAMS	6.6 GRAMS	25.2 GRAMS	528 MILLIGRAMS

EASY SALMON MEATBALLS

	SERVES		PREP TIME		COOK TIME
	2		**5** MINUTES		**25** MINUTES

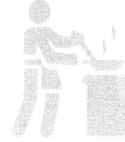

1. Preheat the oven to 350°F.

2. In a large bowl, combine all ingredients. Divide the mixture into 12 meatballs. Apply nonstick cooking spray.

3. Bake for 15-18 minutes.

- **12 ounces** canned pink salmon, drained

- **1/2 cup** whole wheat breadcrumbs

- **2** green onions, finely chopped

- **2 cloves** garlic, minced

- **1/2 tablespoon** grated ginger

- **1** egg

- **1/4 teaspoon** salt

- **1/4 teaspoon** ground black pepper

CALORIES	CARBS	SUGAR	FAT	PROTEIN	SODIUM
198 KCAL	**11.2** GRAMS	**1.0** GRAMS	**5.0** GRAMS	**28.4** GRAMS	**592** MILLIGRAMS

CURRY PEPPER AND FISH

	SERVES 5	PREP TIME 5 MINUTES	COOK TIME 25 MINUTES

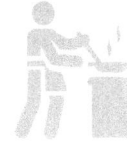

- **17 1/2 ounces** fish fillets
- **2** large onions, sliced
- **1/2** green bell pepper, sliced
- **1/2** red bell pepper, sliced
- **2 cloves** garlic, crushed
- **1 tablespoon** curry powder
- **1 tablespoon** oat bran
- **1 teaspoon** ground cumin seeds
- **1 teaspoon** tomato juice
- **1** bacon stock cube
- **1 cup** water
- **1 pinch** of black pepper

1. Add onions, bell pepper, garlic and tomato juice to a non-stick pan. Simmer over low heat for 5 minutes.

2. Add curry powder, oat bran and cumin while stirring. Break stock cube into smaller pieces in water and add to the mixture. Simmer to a thick consistency.

3. Place the fish fillet in the pan and cooked for 5 minutes. Sprinkle with black pepper and serve.

CALORIES	CARBS	SUGAR	FAT	PROTEIN	SODIUM
191 KCAL	12.0 GRAMS	4.5 GRAMS	3.5 GRAMS	27.9 GRAMS	292 MILLIGRAMS

ASIAN TUNA STEAK

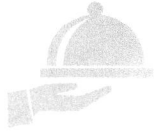

SERVES	PREP TIME	COOK TIME
2	20 MINUTES	10 MINUTES

1. In a large resealable bags, add all ingredients. Massage to mix well. Refrigerate for 15 minutes.

2. Preheat the broiler.

3. Broil for 10-12 minutes, flipping once.

- **6 ounces** tuna steak
- **2 cloves** garlic, minced
- **1 tablespoon** lime juice
- **1/2 tablespoon** low-sodium soy sauce
- **1/2 teaspoon** dark sesame oil
- **1/8 teaspoon** ground black pepper

CALORIES	CARBS	SUGAR	FAT	PROTEIN	SODIUM
112	1.2	0.4	1.9	20.0	145
KCAL	GRAMS	GRAMS	GRAMS	GRAMS	MILLIGRAMS

CRUNCHY FISH FINGERS

SERVES
4

PREP TIME
10
MINUTES

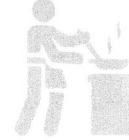

COOK TIME
25
MINUTES

- **1 pound** fish fillets
- **1** large egg
- **1/3 cup** whole-wheat breadcrumbs
- **1/4 cup** grated Parmesan cheese
- **1/2 tablespoon** light butter, melted
- **1/2 teaspoon** dried parsley
- **1/2 teaspoon** paprika
- salt and pepper to taste

1. Preheat oven to 450 degrees.

2. In a smaller dish, beat the egg. In a separate dish, combine the bread crumbs, Parmesan cheese, paprika and parsley.

3. Cut the fish into strips, 3 inches long & 1/2 inches wide.

4. Dip each strip into the egg, then into the crumb mixture.

5. Place the fish strips on a lightly greased baking sheet.

6. Drizzle the melted butter over the fish.

7. Bake for 7-10 minutes, or until fish flakes easily with a fork or knife.

CALORIES	CARBS	SUGAR	FAT	PROTEIN	SODIUM
188	7.9	0.1	5.0	26.0	169
KCAL	GRAMS	GRAMS	GRAMS	GRAMS	MILLIGRAMS

GARLICKY SALMON STEAK

	SERVES		PREP TIME		COOK TIME
	4		**5** MINUTES		**30** MINUTES

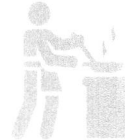

1. Rinse fillet with 1/2 cup milk. To remove fishy odor or taste, you can let it set in milk for up to 5 minutes. Preheat oven to 350 degrees.

2. In a skillet, melt butter and oil until hot. Add in minced garlic.

3. Place in fish, skin side down, and brown for 1 minute. Dust flesh side of fish with garlic salt and lemon pepper. Flip and brown for another minute.

4. Place fish skin side down in pan, transfer entire pan to oven pre-heated at 350 degrees.

5. Roast for 5 minutes per inch of fillet thickness for medium-cooked fish, and 10 minutes per inch for well-done fish.

- **1** large salmon fillet, pan-sized
- **3 cloves** garlic (you can use more or less garlic)
- **1/2 cup** skim milk
- **1 tablespoon** butter
- **1 tablespoon** olive oil
- **1/2-1 teaspoon** lemon pepper
- **1/2 teaspoon** garlic salt

CALORIES	CARBS	SUGAR	FAT	PROTEIN	SODIUM
186 KCAL	**1.0** GRAMS	**0.0** GRAMS	**3.5** GRAMS	**17.2** GRAMS	**50** MILLIGRAMS

CAJUN WHITE FISH

SERVES
2

PREP TIME
5
MINUTES

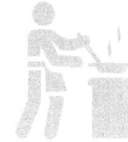

COOK TIME
30
MINUTES

- **2** (6 ounce) white fish fillets
- **1/2 tablespoon** unsalted butter
- **1 teaspoon** paprika
- **1/2 teaspoon** dried thyme
- **1/2 teaspoon** dried oregano
- **1/2 teaspoon** black pepper
- **1/4 teaspoon** garlic salt
- **1/8 teaspoon** cayenne pepper

1. Preheat oven to 400 °F.

2. Sprinkle all spices and herbs over 3 thawed fish fillets.

3. Place the fish fillets on a non-stick baking sheet.

4. Spread the butter on each fish fillet.

5. Cover the entire pan with aluminum foil and set to bake for approximately 25 minutes or until the fish fillets are flaky.

CALORIES	CARBS	SUGAR	FAT	PROTEIN	SODIUM
159	**1.0**	**0.0**	**5.0**	**21.0**	**305**
KCAL	GRAMS	GRAMS	GRAMS	GRAMS	MILLIGRAMS

WHITE FISH IN MEDITERRANEAN SAUCE

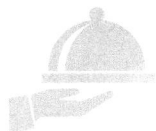

	SERVES 4		PREP TIME 15 MINUTES		COOK TIME 30 MINUTES

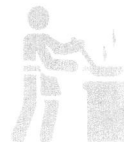

1. Preheat the oven to 425°F.

2. Season the fish with salt and pepper. Place the fish on a baking dish. Set aside.

3. Sauté garlic and onion until fragrant. Then add tomatoes and cook until tender. Add capers, olives, wine, oregano and basil. Reduce to low heat. Stir in cheese. Cook on low until the sauce reduces by half.

4. Spread the sauce on the fish. Bake for 10-15 minutes.

- **1 pound** white fish fillet
- **5** plum tomatoes, diced
- **1/2 cup** chopped onion
- **2 cloves** garlic, minced
- **4 tablespoons** capers
- **6** black olives, pitted and chopped
- **1/4 cup** dry white wine
- **3 tablespoons** fat-free parmesan cheese
- **1/2 teaspoon** dried basil
- pinch of dried oregano

CALORIES	CARBS	SUGAR	FAT	PROTEIN	SODIUM
196 KCAL	7.6 GRAMS	3.6 GRAMS	2.6 GRAMS	29.6 GRAMS	680 MILLIGRAMS

BROCCOLI AND FISH CASSEROLE

	SERVES 3		PREP TIME 5 MINUTES		COOK TIME 40 MINUTES

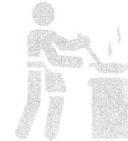

- **1/2 pound** white fish, or about 6 fillets

- **5 ounces** Broccoli frozen

- **1/2 cup** canned mushrooms

- **1/4 cup** Low-fat Mozzarella cheese

- Salt and pepper

1. Layer the broccoli in the bottom of a sprayed baking dish, then spread the mushrooms on top of the broccoli.

2. Place the seasoned fish on top of the mushrooms. Sprinkle generously with mozzarella cheese.

3. Bake the fish fillets at 350 degrees for 35 minutes or until the fillets are crispy or flaky.

CALORIES	CARBS	SUGAR	FAT	PROTEIN	SODIUM
145 KCAL	4.3 GRAMS	2.0 GRAMS	2.8 GRAMS	25.6 GRAMS	273.1 MILLIGRAMS

PORK AND CELERY STIR FRY

	SERVES 2		PREP TIME 10 MINUTES		COOK TIME 20 MINUTES

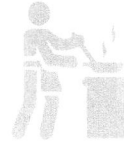

1. In a small bowl, mix the soy sauce and corn starch. Add stock and set aside.

2. Add the oil in wok or non-stick pan over high heat. Add ginger and garlic and cook for 30 second. Add the celery and onions and sauté briefly until slightly softened. Remove the vegetables.

3. Sauté the pork until brown. Add sauce and cook until thickened. Stir continuously. Add vegetables and tomatoes and stir well. Cover and heat for 1 minutes. Serve immediately.

- **7 ounces** lean boneless pork, visible fat removed, thinly sliced
- **2 stalks** celery, sliced
- **3** spring onions, chopped
- **2** tomatoes, cut into wedges
- **2 ounces** fat-free beef stock
- **1 clove** garlic
- **1/2 tablespoon** low-sodium soy sauce
- **1 teaspoon** corn starch
- **1/2 teaspoon** olive oil
- **1/2 teaspoon** grated ginger

CALORIES	CARBS	SUGAR	FAT	PROTEIN	SODIUM
166 KCAL	7.6 GRAMS	3.4 GRAMS	3.8 GRAMS	25.0 GRAMS	580 MILLIGRAMS

GARLIC AND LIME PORK CHOP

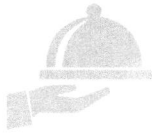

	SERVES		PREP TIME		COOK TIME
	4		**20** MINUTES		**10** MINUTES

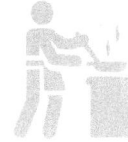

- 2 (6-ounces each) lean boneless pork chops
- **2 cloves** garlic, crushed
- **1/2 teaspoon** kosher salt
- **1/4 teaspoon** pepper
- **1/4 teaspoon** cumin
- **1/4 teaspoon** paprika
- **1/4 teaspoon** chilli powder
- **1/4** lime, juice only
- **1/2 teaspoon** lime zest

1. In a large bowl, mix all ingredient and stir well. Refrigerate for at least 20 minutes to marinate.

2. Preheat the oven and set it to broiler

3. Line broiler with foil and place the pork on top. Broil for 4-5 minutes for each side or until brown

CALORIES	CARBS	SUGAR	FAT	PROTEIN	SODIUM
112 KCAL	**0.9** GRAMS	**0.0** GRAMS	**3.0** GRAMS	**19.0** GRAMS	**184** MILLIGRAMS

DIJON HERBS LAMB CHOPS

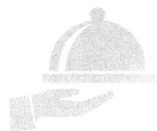

	SERVES 3		PREP TIME 10 MINUTES		COOK TIME 20 MINUTES

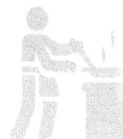

1. Preheat the oven to 375°F.

2. Spread out the herbs on a large plate. Cover the lamp chop with mustard evenly. Coat the lamp chops in herbs.

3. Roast for about 15-20 minutes

- **3 (4-ounces each) lean lamb chops**
- **1 tablespoon** Dijon Mustard
- **2 tablespoons** chopped parsley
- **2 tablespoons** chopped rosemary
- **1 tablespoon** oregano, crumbled
- **1/2 teaspoon** salt
- **1/4 teaspoon** pepper

CALORIES	CARBS	SUGAR	FAT	PROTEIN	SODIUM
134 KCAL	1.2 GRAMS	0.1 GRAMS	4.6 GRAMS	18.6 GRAMS	320 MILLIGRAMS

CHINESE PORK AND SHRIMPS SALAD

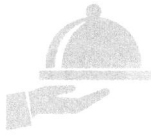

	SERVES		PREP TIME		COOK TIME
	2		**5** MINUTES		**25** MINUTES

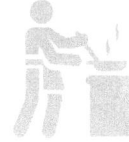

- **4 ounces** pork tenderloin, cooked and shredded

- **2 ounces** shrimps, cooked and chopped

- **2** rice papers

- **2 ounces** bean sprouts, cooked

- **1 tablespoon** fresh basil leaves, chopped

- **1 tablespoon** fresh mint, chopped

- **1/2 tablespoon** lemon juice

1. Evenly divide the meat and vegetable on each rice paper.

2. Squeeze lemon juice on top then roll up.

CALORIES	CARBS	SUGAR	FAT	PROTEIN	SODIUM
101 KCAL	**5.9** GRAMS	**1.7** GRAMS	**1.3** GRAMS	**19.5** GRAMS	**161** MILLIGRAMS

CUCUMBER NOODLES WITH SPICY PAPAYA SAUCE

	SERVES		PREP TIME		COOK TIME
	4		20 MINUTES		20 MINUTES

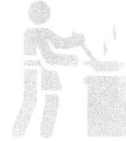

1. In a small bowl, combine soy sauce, hot sauce, oyster sauce, Truvia, salt and 1/2 cup water.

2. Spray a non-stick pan, sauté cucumber noodles over medium heat until slightly softened. Set aside.

3. Sauté spring onions, ginger, onions and pork until pork is brown. Add in the sauce and cook for 10 minutes. Stirring occasionally.

4. Pour the mixture on the noodle. Sprinkle the shredded carrot on top and serve.

- 3 medium seedless cucumber, spiralized
- **12 ounces** extra lean ground pork
- **4** spring onions, finely chopped
- **1** small carrots, shredded
- **1/2** medium onion, cut into strips
- **2 tablespoons** minced fresh ginger
- **2 tablespoons** dark soy sauce
- **1 tablespoon** hot sauce
- **1 tablespoon** oyster sauce
- 1/2 teaspoon Truvia

CALORIES	CARBS	SUGAR	FAT	PROTEIN	SODIUM
182 KCAL	13.6 GRAMS	3.4 GRAMS	4.6 GRAMS	20.6 GRAMS	518 MILLIGRAMS

TRADITIONAL PORK MEATBALLS

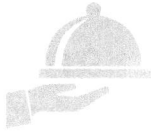

SERVES **4**	**PREP TIME** **10** **MINUTES**	**COOK TIME** **35** **MINUTES**

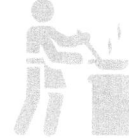

- **1 pound** extra lean ground pork

- **1** egg

- **1/2 cup** whole wheat breadcrumbs, crushed

- **1/4 cup** low sugar/salt ketchup

- **3 tablespoons** stevia (brown sugar blend)

- **1 tablespoon** onion flakes

- **1 teaspoon** dry mustard

- **1/2 teaspoon** salt

- **1/4 teaspoon** ground pepper

- Nonstick Cooking Spray

1. Preheat the oven to 375°F

2. In a small bowl, mix ketchup, stevia and dry mustard. In a large bowl, combine pork, onion flakes, breadcrumbs, salt, pepper, egg and 2 tablespoons of the ketchup mixture.

3. Spray muffin tin with Nonstick Cooking Spray. Divide the meat under 8 portions and roll into balls. Brush the remaining ketchup mixture on top of each meatball.

4. Bake for 30 minutes or until brown.

CALORIES	CARBS	SUGAR	FAT	PROTEIN	SODIUM
258	**22.2**	**6.0**	**7.6**	**26.2**	**558**
KCAL	GRAMS	GRAMS	GRAMS	GRAMS	MILLIGRAMS

SCALLOPS IN TROPICAL SAUCE

	SERVES	PREP TIME	COOK TIME
	4	5 MINUTES	10 MINUTES

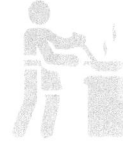

1. Blend papaya, bell pepper, onion, lime juice, cilantro and jalapeño briefly to remove large chunks.

2. In another bowl, mix scallops, flour, salt and pepper evenly.

3. Over medium heat, cook the scallops until golden. Serve the scallops on the papaya sauce.

- **1 pound** sea scallops
- **1** small papaya, peeled, seeded and chopped
- **1** red bell pepper, chopped
- **1/2** red onion, chopped
- **2 tablespoons** all-purpose flour
- **2 tablespoons** fresh lime juice
- **1 tablespoon** chopped cilantro
- **1 tablespoon** olive oil
- **1 teaspoon** minced jalapeño peppers
- **1 dash** of salt

CALORIES	CARBS	SUGAR	FAT	PROTEIN	SODIUM
172 KCAL	12.5 GRAMS	4.3 GRAMS	4.4 GRAMS	38.0 GRAMS	346 MILLIGRAMS

SHRIMP SCAMPI

	SERVES 2		PREP TIME 5 MINUTES		COOK TIME 10 MINUTES

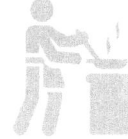

- **6 ounces** uncooked shrimp, peeled
- **1 teaspoon** olive oil
- **1** medium green onion, diced
- **1/2 tablespoon** lemon juice
- **1/2 tablespoon** Parmesan cheese
- **1/4 teaspoon** basil
- **1/4 teaspoon** salt
- **1/8 teaspoon** garlic powder

1. In a medium skillet, heat oil over medium high heat.

2. Add shrimp and other ingredients. Cook 3-7 minutes depending on the size of shrimp.

3. Remove from heat; sprinkle with Parmesan cheese.

CALORIES	CARBS	SUGAR	FAT	PROTEIN	SODIUM
124 KCAL	2.0 GRAMS	0.1 GRAMS	4.5 GRAMS	18.1 GRAMS	310 MILLIGRAMS

GRANNY'S CRAB CAKES

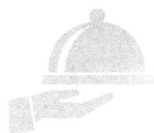 SERVES
·

PREP TIME
·
MINUTES

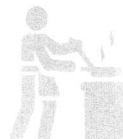 COOK TIME
·
MINUTES

1. In a medium bowl, Combine all ingredients. Divide the mixture into 8 portions and shape into 1/2-inch thick patties.

2. Spray a non-stick pan and heat over medium heat. Add the crab cake and cook for 3 minutes then flip and cooked for another 3 minutes or until golden brown.

- 1 pound lump crab meat
- 1/2 cup whole wheat breadcrumbs
- 1/2 cup almond flour
- 1/4 cup corn meal
- 1 jalapeno pepper, seeded and chopped
- 3 tablespoons chopped scallion
- 2 tablespoons liquid egg whites
- 2 tablespoons lemon juice
- 2 tablespoons fat-free plain yogurt
- 1/2 teaspoon paprika
- 1/2 teaspoon salt
- Nonstick Cooking Spray

CALORIES	CARBS	SUGAR	FAT	PROTEIN	SODIUM
238	18.4	1.4	7.6	27.0	672
KCAL	GRAMS	GRAMS	GRAMS	GRAMS	MILLIGRAMS

SHIRATAKI FETTUCCINE WITH SHRIMPS

SERVES 3

PREP TIME 5 MINUTES

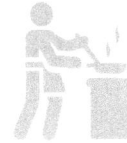

COOK TIME 20 MINUTES

- **1 pound** peeled shrimp

- **8 ounces** Shirataki Fettuccine noodles

- **1/2 cup** white wine

- **1 1/2 tablespoons** Extra Virgin Olive Oil

- **1 tablespoon** of crushed red peppers

- **2 teaspoons** of minced garlic

- **1/2 teaspoon** salt

- **1/4 teaspoon** pepper

1. Drain Shirataki noodles. Rinse noodles under cool water. Drain and squeeze out excess water as much as possible.

2. In a non-stick skillet, mix the shrimp, oil, pepper, and garlic. Cook until shrimp is pink. Make sure the shrimp is not overcooked or hardened.

3. During the last two minutes of cooking time, add the wine and let evaporate.

4. Toss shrimp mixture with noodles and serve.

CALORIES	CARBS	SUGAR	FAT	PROTEIN	SODIUM
316	6.0	0.0	9.8	31.4	396
KCAL	GRAMS	GRAMS	GRAMS	GRAMS	MILLIGRAMS

SHRIMP CEVICHE

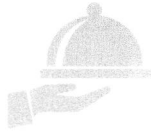

	SERVES		PREP TIME		COOK TIME
	2		**15** MINUTES		**10** MINUTES

1. In a bowl, mix the shrimp and lime juice.

2. Cover and let sit for about 10 to 15 minutes or until the color turns to pink. Do not marinate too long, as the shrimp will "overcook" and harden.

3. Add the onions, tomatoes, chili peppers and cilantro.

4. Gently stir to combine.

5. Season with salt and serve cold.

- **1/2 pound** medium raw shrimp

- **1/2 cup** lime juice

- **2** medium tomatoes diced or 4 ounces canned, diced tomatoes

- **1/2** small red onion, peeled and chopped

- **1 bunch** cilantro, stemmed and chopped

- **1** serrano chili peppers, ribs and seeds removed, minced

CALORIES	CARBS	SUGAR	FAT	PROTEIN	SODIUM
160 KCAL	**13.0** GRAMS	**5.0** GRAMS	**1.0** GRAMS	**25.0** GRAMS	**265** MILLIGRAMS

SEARED SCALLOPS IN WINE SAUCE

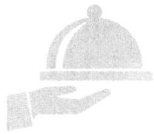

	SERVES		PREP TIME		COOK TIME
	2		**10** MINUTES		**15** MINUTES

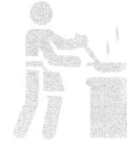

- **12 ounces** sea scallops, dried

- **1/2 teaspoon** olive oil

- **1/4 cup** dry white wine

- **1/2 tablespoon** balsamic vinegar

- **1/2 tablespoon** chopped fresh parsley

- **1/2 tablespoon** chopped fresh chives

- **1/4 teaspoon** salt

- **1/8 teaspoon** pepper

- Nonstick Cooking Spray

1. Add oil to a non-stick pan, sear scallops for 3 minutes each side or until golden. Set aside.

2. Add white wine, vinegar, all herbs and seasoning to the pan. Heat until bubbly. Toss in the scallops and stir quickly. Serve immediately.

CALORIES	CARBS	SUGAR	FAT	PROTEIN	SODIUM
166 KCAL	**3.0** GRAMS	**1.0** GRAMS	**2.6** GRAMS	**25.6** GRAMS	**580** MILLIGRAMS

SALAD TOMATOES CUPS

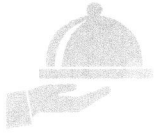

	SERVES		PREP TIME		COOK TIME
	2		35 MINUTES		0 MINUTES

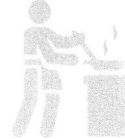

1. In a medium bowl, combine shrimp, celery, shallots, basil, mayonnaise and vinegar. Season with salt and pepper.

2. Spoon the mixture into the tomatoes. Garnish with pinch of paprika and serve.

- **1/2 pound** shrimp, peeled, deveined, cooked and chopped

- **2** large ripe tomatoes, cored

- **1/2 stalk** celery, chopped

- **1** shallot, minced

- **2 tablespoons** chopped fresh basil

- **1 tablespoon** low-fat mayonnaise

- **1/2 tablespoon** white wine vinegar

- salt and pepper to taste

- pinch of paprika

CALORIES	CARBS	SUGAR	FAT	PROTEIN	SODIUM
160 KCAL	9.0 GRAMS	5.6 GRAMS	2.6 GRAMS	25.8 GRAMS	618 MILLIGRAMS

BROCCOLI FRITTERS

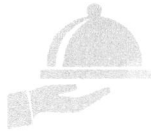

	SERVES		PREP TIME		COOK TIME
	1		**5** MINUTES		**10** MINUTES

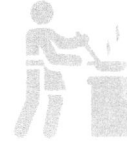

- **1 cup** chopped broccoli, finely chopped and cooked

- **1/2 cup** fat-free mozzarella cheese

- **2 tablespoons** low-fat parmesan cheese

- **3 tablespoons** liquid egg whites

- **1 1/2 teaspoons** flax seed meal

- **1 teaspoon** light Italian dressing

- **1/8 teaspoon** garlic powder

- **1/8 teaspoon** ground pepper

- Nonstick Cooking Spray

1. In a large bowl, combine all ingredients.

2. Divide the mixture into 2 portions and shape into patties.

3. Spray a non-stick pan. Heat the patties for 5 minutes over low/medium heat until brown. Flip and heat for another 5 minutes.

CALORIES	CARBS	SUGAR	FAT	PROTEIN	SODIUM
206 KCAL	**16.6** GRAMS	**2.0** GRAMS	**7.2** GRAMS	**20.8** GRAMS	**616** MILLIGRAMS

SPICED TOFU SCRAMBLE

	SERVES		PREP TIME		COOK TIME
	1		**15** MINUTES		**15** MINUTES

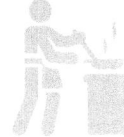

1. Roll the tofu in a clean towel and place a heavy subject on top for 15 minutes.

2. In a small bowl, mix the spice with 2 tablespoons of water.

3. Sauté the onion and bell peppers over medium heat until softened. Add kale and cover for 2 minutes. Season with salt and pepper.

4. Put the tofu into 1-inch cube.

5. Move the veggie to the side. Add the tofu and sauté for 2 minutes. Then add 3/4 of the sauce over the tofu and the remaining over the veggie. Mix well and cook for another 5-7 minutes.

- **8 ounces** extra firm tofu
- **2 cups** kale, loosely chopped
- **1/2** red pepper, thinly sliced
- **1/4** red onion, thinly sliced
- **1/2 teaspoon** sea salt
- **1/2 teaspoon** garlic powder
- **1/2 teaspoon** cumin powder
- **1/4 teaspoon** chilli powder
- **1/4 teaspoon** turmeric
- Nonstick Cooking Spray

CALORIES	CARBS	SUGAR	FAT	PROTEIN	SODIUM
206 KCAL	**17.4** GRAMS	**0.4** GRAMS	**4.4** GRAMS	**21.4** GRAMS	**190** MILLIGRAMS

Nutrition Information Summary

	Calories (kCal)	Carbs (g)	Sugar (g)	Fat (g)	Protein (g)	Sodium (mg)
Grilled Lemongrass Beef	124	3.6	0.1	3.8	18.3	182
Mustard Beef Lettuce Wrap	155	5.8	2.5	3.8	21	227
Beef and Veggies Stir Fry	198	9.2	3.8	5.2	26.8	674
Quick Taco and Beans Soup	216	29.2	2.8	2.2	20	536
One-pan Mexican Beef	204	8.8	3.8	5.4	26.4	678
Greek Spinach Chicken Salad	180	11.8	6.2	6	27.6	452
Ranch Chicken Salad	126	10	5.6	3.4	20.2	630
Lentil Turkey Sausage	192	19.2	1.8	2.6	22.2	392
Herb-Roasted Chicken	105	0.5	0	4.5	16.6	315
Spicy Citrus Chicken Stir Fry	98	0.5	0.1	3.4	16.6	239
Chicken Fajita	134	4.1	0.9	3.3	22.7	375
Traditional Turkey Sausage	158	1.6	0	8.2	22.2	380
Chicken and Peas Stir Fry	118	3.4	1.2	0.6	23	236
Caprese Chicken	306	5.4	2.4	8	44	140
White Bean and Chicken Soup	160	16	1.6	2.2	20.2	610
Chicken and Avocado Lettuce Wraps	216	10.6	3.2	9.2	23.6	542
Turkey Satay	126	18.4	3.7	5.4	3.4	406
lemon and Thyme Chicken	110	2	0.4	0.4	22.6	112
Spinach Feta Stuffed Chicken	166	4.2	1.6	1.2	30	656
Fool-proof Salsa Chicken	184	11	8	0.4	24	592
Pinto Bean Turkey Enchilada	288	21	0	9.6	22.8	650
Pomodoro Chicken with Squash	182	9.5	0.9	2.6	18.5	452

	Calories (kCal)	Carbs (g)	Sugar (g)	Fat (g)	Protein (g)	Sodium (mg)
Chicken Basque with Zucchini Noodle	113	8.6	5.9	2.6	18.9	372
Thai Chicken Zoodles	141	6.8	3.6	4.8	20.1	363
Hawaiian Tuna Poke	182	2	0	4.8	29.4	620
Tuna Salad Lettuce Wraps	95	4.8	1.8	1.4	17.3	388
Curry Spiced Salmon Steak	160	1.8	0	1.8	36.4	512
Simple Rainbow Trout	240	10	0	5	25	338
Tuna Cake	160	8	0	2	24	480
Dijon Lemon Orange Roughy	228	6	0	8	34	314
Lemony Tilapia	121	1.3	0.3	4.3	20.1	282.3
Spicy Citrus Tilapia	134	25.3	3.4	1.5	0.3	294
Broiled Citrus Salmon	166	3.6	0.4	1.6	37.4	264
Salmon and Egg Scramble	194	2.8	0.8	7.8	26.2	640
Italian Tilapia Alfredo	168	11.6	3.6	4.2	22.6	648
Cheesy Spicy Halibut	136	7.6	0.6	1	25	540
Mackerel cakes	204	9.6	1.2	6.6	25.2	528
Easy Salmon Meatballs	198	11.2	1	5	28.4	592
Curry Pepper and Fish	191	12	4.5	3.5	27.9	292
Asian Tuna Steak	112	1.2	0.4	1.9	20	145
Crunchy Fish Fingers	188	7.9	0.1	5	26	169.4
Garlicky Salmon steak	186	1	0	3.5	17.2	49.7
Cajun White Fish	159	1	0	5	21	305
White Fish in Mediterranean Sauce	196	7.6	3.6	2.6	29.6	680
Broccoli and Fish Casserole	145	4.3	2	2.8	25.6	273.1
Pork and Celery Stir Fry	166	7.6	3.4	3.8	25	580

	Calories (kCal)	Carbs (g)	Sugar (g)	Fat (g)	Protein (g)	Sodium (mg)
Garlic and Lime Pork Chops	112	0.9	0	3	19	184
Dijon Herbs Lamb Chops	134	1.2	0.1	4.6	18.6	320
Vietnamese Pork and Shrimps Spring Rolls	101	5.9	1.7	1.3	19.5	161
Cucumber Noodles with Spicy Pork	182	13.6	3.4	4.6	20.6	518
Traditional Pork Meatballs	258	22.2	6	7.6	26.2	558
Scallops in Tropical Sauce	172	12.5	4.3	4.4	38	346
Shrimp Scampi	124	2	0.1	4.5	18.1	310
Granny's Crab Cakes	238	18.4	1.4	7.6	27	672
Shirataki Fettuccine with Shrimps	316	6	0	9.8	31.4	396
Shrimp Ceviche	160	13	5	1	25	265
Traditional Seared Scallops in Wine sauce	166	3	1	2.6	25.6	580
Salad Tomatoes Cups	160	9	5.6	2.6	25.8	618
Broccoli Fritters	206	16.6	2	7.2	20.8	616
Spiced Tofu Scramble	206	17.4	0.4	4.4	21.4	190

THANK YOU FOR READING!

We hope this book has provide you some new inspiration. Thank you again for picking up our book and going through it.

STELLA LAYNE & SELENA LANCASTER 2017

Made in the USA
Coppell, TX
30 October 2021